EXCAVATIONS
Twenty Oedipal Prose Poems

By
Harold Wolfe

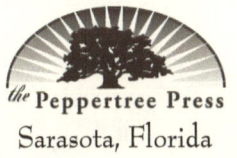

the Peppertree Press
Sarasota, Florida

ISBN: 978-0-9821654-4-7

Library of Congress Number: 2008939820

Printed in the U.S.A.

Printed November 2008

~ For Sherry ~

And for

Irving Schneider, M.D.

Julian Barish, M.D.

Christine Svenson, ARNP

About the Author

Harold Wolfe was born in Binghamton, N.Y., in 1926 and served in the United States Army from 1944 to 1946.

After graduation from Hartwick College in Oneonta, N.Y., he married Sherry Siegel of Brooklyn, N.Y. They have two sons, fourteen grandchildren and eight great-grandchildren.

Before retiring in November 1991, he worked fifteen years as a medical editor-writer and public information officer for several federal health agencies, including the National Institutes of Health, and twenty-four years as press secretary for two commissioners of mental health and six chief administrative judges in New York State.

Since 1988, he has written eighty poems. Since 1992, the Sarasota Herald-Tribune has published eighty-one of his letters to the editor and seven guest columns. His play "The Burning" was performed at the Manatee Players Riverfront Theatre in Bradenton, Florida, as part of their 2005 New Play Festival.

He has also performed in two musicals and a play at the Players Theatre of Sarasota: "Fiddler on the Roof" (1993), "Rags" (1994), and "Twilight of the Golds" (1997).

CONTENTS

INTRODUCTION

Most of my adult life I have had a special interest in the "unconscious," which is the hidden part of mental activity that does not ordinarily enter the individual's awareness.

I have also been particularly interested in what psychodynamic psychiatry and psychology call "unconscious motivation," that is, the drives, such as repressed wishes, that are unknown to the individual who harbors them, but can be revealed during psychotherapy.

But most of all, I have had an abiding curiosity about the role of the Oedipus Complex, especially its derivative neuroses, in shaping or misshaping human lives.

The word "Oedipus," Greek for "swollen foot," entered western culture about 2,000 years before Freud ever started writing about the Oedipus Complex. But Freud, steeped in the classics, surely read *Oedipus Rex*, the world's first great tragedy.

Written by the Greek dramatist Sophocles, it tells the story of Oedipus, the son of King Laius of Thebes and Queen Jacosta, who is raised by a shepherd foster parent and in fulfillment of an oracle, unknowingly kills his father and marries his mother. Upon learning the truth about his horrible crimes, Oedipus blinds himself.

In other words, upon becoming aware of his crimes, Oedipus cripples himself. That is exactly what I had in mind when I said above that an Oedipal neurosis can misshape human lives.

Freud's work and the work of many of his followers taught us that the images the unconscious mind creates, especially forbidden fantasies, wishes and hatreds, inexorably find an exit. They tunnel their way up into life, including art and literature.

Sophocles was a human being and had a childhood. And I suggest that his first great family-triangle tragedy, while derived in part from Greek myths, was also rooted in his inner life, that is, in his unconscious. And not merely in *his* unconscious, but, I dare say, in what Carl Jung, one of Freud's leading progeny, called the "collective unconscious" of humankind.

To put it another way, Sophocles did not simply dream up *Oedipus Rex*. His unconscious mind did, and his conscious imagination and pen were his hammer and chisel. Using that same process, I say modestly, I created my Oedipal poems. And so have thousands of other poets, writers and artists, whether they were aware of it or not.

What exactly is the Oedipus Complex? According to Webster's, it comprises "the positive libidinal feelings of a child toward the parent of the opposite sex and the hostile or jealous feelings toward the parent of the same sex that may be a source of adult personality disorder when unresolved" or, I would add, resolved malignantly.

When it occurs in a female, it is called the Electra Complex after another mythical Greek, Electra, a sister of Orestes who helps him kill their mother, Clytemnestra, for committing adultery and killing their father, King Agamemnon of Mycenae and leader of the Greeks in the Trojan War.

For those who wish to explore this subject further, I recommend two fine works. The first is *Freud: A Life for Our Time,* by Peter Gay, one of Freud's major biographers, who calls the Oedipus Complex the "nuclear complex of the neuroses." The second excellent book on the subject, especially on developmental psychology, is *Identity and the Life Cycle*, by Erik Erikson. Erikson taught that the guilt that is at the center of the Oedipal neuroses "may find expression in a self-restriction which keeps an individual from living up to his or her inner capacities." Or, I must add, which cripples their ability to work and love productively and happily.

Psychoanalysts and developmental psychologists are not the only source of knowledge about the unconscious and its powerful role in shaping or misshaping human behavior. Some of our finest writers and poets, untrained in science but rich in learning from life and suffering, also have been driven to unconsciously probe and transform into art what the American scholar, teacher, and former Librarian of Congress Daniel J. Boorstin has called, in his book *The Creators,* the "wilderness within" which, I think you will agree, is a beautiful metaphor for the unconscious.

And I am sure that those who've read a lot have found other references or allusions to the unconscious, or the "wilderness within," or its counterpart, "the child within," in the novels of such writers as the American

Lillian Smith, who had a special interest in Freud and American psychiatrists like Karl Menninger.

Or in the works of two British novelists quoted by Boorstin: D.H. Lawrence, who wrote "the best we can do is try to hold ourselves in unison with the deeps which are inside us." And Virginia Woolf, who imagined "the world that lies submerged in the depths of our unconscious being."

The prose poems that follow are, to a great extent, rooted in my own personal lifetime struggle for psychological wholeness or integrity. Thus, almost all of the poems are autobiographical. All the dreams and fantasies are true. I dreamt them; I fantasized them.

But several poems, particularly the disturbing "The Bum" and "The Drunk," are wholly the product of my research and my imagination and describe the worst consequences of an untreated, or poorly treated, crippling Oedipal neurosis.

And now, let the poems begin.

Excavations
Twenty Oedipal Prose Poems

I

Wonder

A seed dropped in the earth becomes a rose
that nourishes souls thirsting for beauty.

Another planted seed becomes an elm
beneath whose boughs is found repose.

Still another seed, a human seed,
is planted in a mother's warmth,
emerges as a child, becomes a boy, then a man
who struggles to make poetry from prose
and paint with words the wondrous miracles of life.

II

The Stuff of Poetry

What a burden it is, but what a blessing still
to be able to feel keenly, like a naked nerve,
all the pains as well as joys of being human.
It is the stuff of poetry.

So let life sometimes rage, pour anguish down on me.
I'll still exult, because I am and because of poetry.

III

Roots

These things are clear to me now.

That as the oak must sway
before the raging winds of nature,
so I must bend before the storms
that swirl deep within my inner life.

That as a poet, I am compelled to tell
a tale arising from my early memories,
my dreams, my fantasies.

That many poems of mine are rooted in past feelings,
feelings of the injured child that still resides in me,
feelings that still work their way into my daily life,
feelings to which I must give written form, continually,
in order to preserve the soundness of my searching mind.

IV

Hidden Feelings

Hidden feelings are no mystery to me,
for my poetic musings allow me to explore
the demoned caverns of my mind
evermore, evermore, evermore.

V

Demons

Like an undertow that threatens
to drag him out to sea,
demons lurking deep within his mind
conspire to pull him back to childhood,
where, small and weak and defenseless,
he cannot challenge the dominance of his sire
and so escapes the danger of severe punishment.

VI

First Session

When we first met, fear lurked,
like a tiger, behind my eyes.
Helplessness enveloped me like a lead net.
Close to hopelessness, I stood
at the edge of an abyss,
looking down at nothingness,
wanting only to escape
the terror that was nearly paralyzing me.

VII

The Digger

He digs in the coal pits of the mind.
Picks and shovels, then uncovers
primal urges: coupling, killing;
evil wishes, incestuous and patricidal;
fluctuating filial love and hate,
and the rending, sometimes crippling,
tugs of war that they engender.

All this labor leaves the digger aching,
choking on the dust and, without warning, sobbing.

VIII

For Irving

What have we two wrought
in the quiet of this room?

A heart was torn open,
and a mind unchained.

IX

For Julian

I am on course again, O pilot mine,
though I sail on a stormy sea.

And I will suffer any pain
to continue to be free.

And free, by heaven, I will be.
No reef, no shoal shall obstruct me.

X

Farewell, Farewell,
O Pilot Mine

Farewell, farewell, O pilot mine.
The seas that we have tandem sailed
call out, call out to me,
"Alone, alone, your time has come
to venture forth alone."

Farewell, farewell, O pilot mine.
The crashing waves, the roaring winds,
not so fearful anymore,
call out, call out to me,
"Alone, alone, you have the strength
to risk the deep alone."

Farewell, farewell, O pilot mine.
The white stars in the ebon sky
call out, call out to me,
"Alone, alone, the man you struggled
to become can now sail on alone."

XI

Beginnings

She was the sea that gave me life.

She was the stream that first nourished me.

She was the cove that first sheltered me from storms.

She was the sun that first brightened my days.

She was the beauty that shaped my first thoughts of love.

And now she dwells deep within my heart.

XII

She Once Was
Young and Beautiful

She once was young and beautiful
and the men in her life adored her,
adored her olive skin and auburn hair,
her dark brown eyes and seashell ears,
her smiling mouth, from which emerged
an endless string of melodies
that echo still in my joyful memories.

XIII

Mother and Son

I saw a mother and her young son
sitting in a cool New York City subway car
on a hot and muggy August day.

Her queenly face, chiseled out of flawless ebony,
caught and held my gaze.
I could not take my eyes off her,
nor could her son.

We were enthralled by her,
by her dark eyes and straight nose,
her wavy black hair and shell-like ears,
her full lips and high cheekbones,
features that could have been passed down
from Ethiopian royalty.

As I look back at that moment
and recall that mother and her son,
I know that common, hidden fantasies
of worship and desire
compelled the two of us, the boy, the man,
to quietly adore her,
and that the man I am saw in him the boy I used to be.

XIV

Woman Is a Sea

Woman is a sea,
waves and depths and spray,
source of life and ecstasy.
Woman, sea,
envelop me.

XV

The Bum

Behind a smiling mask,
the boy feels apprehensive,
as if a tiger's always on the prowl.

He bites his nails down to the quick,
washes hands and counts to three, repeatedly,
is careful not to step on sidewalk cracks.

He finds great pleasure in solo sex,
knows Hollywood beauties in erotic fantasies,
feels guilty, vows not to sin again,
but goes on doing it nightly anyhow.
Falls asleep, wakes up trembling
in the middle of the night,
swears to God he will be good.

The anxious boy, now a man,
grabs the brass ring, panics, flees,
becomes a derelict who sleeps in alleyways
and feeds at the city's cafeteria of garbage cans.

As long as he's a bum,
he's able to feel safe.
The tiger's in its cage.

XVI

The Wounded

Everywhere I walk I see people limping,
stumbling, falling, unseen crutches failing.
They are strangers to life's sweet victories,
victims of oozing wounds deep within their minds,
lesions of guilt and fear that twist men's lives.

XVII

The Drunk

In ragged clothes, unshaven and unwashed,
he holds out a filthy, trembling hand
to passersby for coins to buy
the wine that keeps him numb.

Bleary-eyed, he staggers down
a damp and dreary Bowery street,
reaches down for a cigarette butt,
stumbles, sprawls into a pile
of urine-soaked trash.

On his knees, he moans,
"Jesus, I thought you died for me."

Darkness, bottle emptied, he falls asleep
as rats scurry across the newspapers
in which he's wrapped himself against the cold.

He dreams he walks into Christ's tomb.

XVIII

Shells

The poet walks along the shore
and views the wreckage in the sand:
shells of children once full of wonder,
ready to explore the mysteries of the deep.

But a hurricane engulfed them,
blew the spirit out of them,
dumped them on the beach,
where the poet paints their anguish
on a canvass of compassion,
using brushes dipped in his own agony.

XIX

Encounters

1

I came upon you, my dead father, in a fantasy.
We were seated by a quiet forest pond
that was a glistening metaphor
for the innocence of childhood,
when not a drop of conscious, hostile jealousy
tainted the deep affection that I felt for you.
How unnatural such pure filial love must seem
to those acquainted with the tragedy
of Oedipus the king and all that it implies
for ordinary men as well as royalty.

2

I came upon you, my dead father, in a dream.
We were circling each other in a boxing ring.
Your head was shaved smooth and glistened.
Your face was the face of a heartless brute.
The muscles in your neck and chest, arms and legs,
were the muscles of a predatory beast.
But I overcame my fear and engaged you in combat.

We snarled, stalked, and pummeled each other.
Our mutual hatred exploded.
We reveled in our beastliness.
Our bloody fists beat out our savage fury.
We fought not just to conquer,
but to destroy each other.
Then the dream ended. And I slept.

3

I came upon you, my dead father, in another dream
of heart-pounding, throat-choking hatred.
Now I was the brute, the predatory beast,
and, drained of all humanity, I attacked you as if
you were a suddenly trapped, terrified bully.
Overcome by loathing, engulfed by cruelty,
ignoring your cries for mercy,
I battered you unceasingly.
No part of your body was safe from my rage.
And, as you sank to the ground,
I spat my hatred into your bloody face.
Then the dream ended. And I slept.

4

I came upon you, my dead father,
in yet another dream.
We were seated by the pond
where we first met
in the fantasy that began this poem
of recollection and travail.

I looked into your face,
and you smiled at me
in a way that seemed to say,
as you had never said before,
be strong, be free, be gone.
Then I turned and walked away from you
hand in hand with life.

XX

Excavations

1

It was autumn, the season of showering leaves.
You and I, Father, were standing in a field,
a few miles from home, where the grass was like straw,
and the sky was gray and forbidding.

In that field, as the gray sky gazed down on us,
you carried a shotgun in your pie baker's hands,
hands with which you sometimes patted my head,
once caressed my mother's breasts before my eyes.

Suddenly, you raised the gun and pulled the trigger.
The gun roared, and our beagle, Lady, howled joyfully.
And the roar of the gun, the howl of the happy dog,
but mostly your look of glee frightened and puzzled me.
No rabbit, squirrel, or pheasant died on that autumn day.
But the child that I was felt strange, small, uneasy.

2

It was winter, the season when crisp, cold air
stings the ears and nose.
The ground in the village we were visiting
was blanketed by snow.
The limbs of the pines in the nearby park

23

bowed under their white frosting,
transforming the park into a glistening wonderland.
But you, Father, restless, unable to simply enjoy
the sheer beauty of that glorious winter day,
you picked up your shotgun again,
picked up that instrument of death again
and walked alone into the nearby forest,
beyond the peaceful, sparkling park.

A few minutes later, as I sat on a bench in the park,
the stillness of that quiet winter day
was shattered by the roar of your gun.
A small brown squirrel died by your hands
on that once splendid and tranquil day,
a creature as innocent and harmless as I
died by your hands on that now terrible day.
And the child that I was felt strange, small, anxious.

3

It is now, not a recollected season in the past.
And I descend deep into my mind
in an attempt to confront my self,
confront the truth about my self,
about the innocent, harmless creature me,
the father-worshipping little boy me,
the "I love you, Daddy," pure little boy me.
That boy was expected to be,

or so I thought and, more important, felt,
the only white sheep in our entire family,
was expected to be and do only good
all the time, all the goddamn time,
every goddamn waking minute of every goddamn day,
while all the time inside my self
I hid a rage to rage.
And those unnatural expectations,
my family's and, now I see,
mine as well, mine most of all,
became the felon that stole from me
the treasure of my full humanity.
Yes, I helped forge the chains
that shackled me emotionally,
and I must now explore the reasons why.
I must ask my mind and heart: Why?

4

In my hands, I hold two black-and-white photographs,
two goblets brimming with the wine of childhood memories.
I drink deeply from each of them.
In the first, I am two, and in an act of daring for us both,
you, Father, beaming with pride in your brave little boy,
balance an erect and smiling me in your right hand,
held straight out from your muscular shoulder.
You were that strong. I was that fearless.
In that instant caught on film you said yes to me,

encouraged me to reach out, grab the world, make it mine.
"Yes," I heard you say. "Let the flame of life within you
blaze and roar, son. Scream out to all creation, son,
'I am, I am, I am. I will, I will, I will.'"
And the primal self within me felt secure and courageous.

In the second photograph, I am four,
radiating self-confidence.
Just look at me standing there jauntily,
playing the little man exuberantly,
holding an unlit cigarette, symbol of grownupness,
one of your cigarettes, Father,
and my right foot cocked on its heel, assuredly.
It is a portrait of me as a growing boy,
the seeds of my manhood planted,
my father still saying yes to me.
And the child that I was felt secure and daring.

5

No photograph captured the incident
that I will now relate,
a stab of pain repeated too many times
during the crucial span
that marked my passage from boy to man.
I must rely, then, not on film,
but on painful memories of days gone by.

I was six, or maybe seven, no more I'm sure,
hungry for life, beauty, knowledge,
confident in myself, vigorous,
proud of my budding muscles,
prouder still of my emerging intellect.

One day, Father, when you returned
from your work of baking and delivering pies
to workmen's restaurants around our shoe factory town,
I ran to tell you of my latest victories
in the classroom earlier that day
and afterwards at play.

What was your shocking response,
your stinging no to me?
"Think you're a real big shot, don't you?"
were the words you fired back,
like bullets tearing into my heart.

Father, that searing slap in the face,
if not always in those exact words,
then in equally painful variations,
caused me such deep anguish, shame, and guilt,
on that day and on others,
that I quickly replaced boasts
with feigned humility and so betrayed my self.

6

But now I know, Father —
not only from my explorations of my self,
but from my endless search for knowledge
about the forces that shape human striving,
most of all the need for self-respect —
why you were compelled to put me down, again and again.
And, through that knowing,
I have moved toward healing
and reconciliation with my self and, yes, with you.

Father, poor man, I came to see how you envied
other, better educated, more respected men,
more successful doctors, lawyers, businessmen.
I came to sense that you were riddled
with doubts about your own manhood and accomplishments
and pained by a terrible lack of pride in yourself,
which hunting, fishing, boxing, daily strenuous exercise
at the Y could not supply, no matter how hard you tried.

And so, Father, you transformed me, unknowingly,
the innocent, harmless me, the "I love you, Daddy" me
into one of your competitors, as I had years before,
unconsciously, made you the first of mine.

You had good reason to envy me, Father, if unknowingly.
You had good reason to fear me, if unknowingly.

And I suspect now that you knew it, instinctively.
You see, Father, I have also learned,
through a sometimes agonizing excavation
of my deepest, hidden feelings and forgotten memories,
that the innocent, harmless creature me
was not innocent or harmless at all,
at least not in the deepest cavern of my mind,
which is the lair of all the powerful forces
that shape our lives and destinies.

And so the time has come in this exposing tale of mine,
this backward glance at some events that molded me,
to strip away the masquerade of innocence and harmlessness
that I put on to cover up my natural, but forbidden wishes
and by such revelation, liberate my full humanity.

7

My dear departed father, Joseph Jacob,
whose seed helped give me life,
I know from dreams and fantasies,
from musings and exhumed memories,
that in the early years
of my adventure here on earth,
not only did I perceive but,
more important still,
I keenly felt that there was I,
there was you,

and, in between the two of us,
there was our darling Lillian,
my beautiful mother, your cherished wife.
And in that ancient triangular arrangement,
the hidden war between the two of us was waged,
with not a chance of victory for me.
I also know that if you loved her passionately,
and I do not doubt you did,
then I adored her, too, with no less ardor,
for she was then the entire world to me
and by her love affirmed my being and my worth.

8

I have recalled uncounted times throughout my life,
and will continue to recall till death claims me,
a scene involving her and me that is by far
my happiest boyhood memory.
On our kitchen table, where I sit,
while a cold December wind blows outside,
there is a bowl of hot oatmeal
that she has just prepared,
nourishment for my young, growing body.

Sitting across the table from me,
she holds in her right hand
that school day's list of spelling words,
nourishment for my young, growing intellect.

And as I eat that mother-made mush
with undisguised joy, she calls out to me,
and I spell out unerringly,
much to her delight and mine —
O joy compounding joy —
the words that later on in class
will test my intellect and industry.

9

I soon learned in those early, formative years
how to win my mother's admiration and respect
through such displays of my cerebral gifts,
as modest as they were.

And with the passing of the years,
it came to me in therapy,
my intellect became my sword in the son-and-father war
that raged within our home behind a smokescreen
of excessive son-and-father love.

What I was unaware of then,
but discovered decades later
as I explored my self, was this.
Each time I drew that sword
and scored an intellectual victory,
surpassing my undereducated father cerebrally,
it was as if I had slain him.

That was the innocent, harmless creature me,
the loving son, the adoring son,
like Oedipus, a patricide,
acting out my murderous rage
on the hidden mainstage of my mind.

10

For that crime, the unconscious crime of sons
since the first sons, which I committed again and again,
I paid a bitter price
in agonizing guilt and paralyzing fear
of shameful discovery and painful punishment.

To escape the guilt and fear,
and the feeling of conviction, too,
that I harbored evil, demanding punishment repeatedly,
to escape that web of unimaginable terror,
I condemned myself to fail from time to time
by disqualifying myself, as if to execute myself
again and again; or failing that, to nearly drown
in a torrent of crippling anxiety,
and then, upon recovering with the passage of time,
begin the cycle all over again.
But there was no escape, at least not then.

11

I could not help myself in those young manhood years.
But then, thanks to therapy and the healing that it brought,
I began to dare to hope I could prevail.
My inner, primal self, the "I" in me, cried out,
and still cries out, "I can, I can, I know I can!"

I sigh now that my story has been told,
the truth about me bared, my full humanity revealed.
And so, with thanks for all the blessings rained down on me,
I lay aside the work of digging up old, hidden memories
and search instead for challenges that are more real
to occupy my life, my mind, my zeal.

Harold Wolfe ~ 2008